Keto Bread

92 recipes to lose weight fast with easy step-by-step bread recipes. The ultimate Low-carb keto diet bread cookbook.

Sarah Foster

Table of Contents

Introduction

I want to thank you and congratulate you for purchasing the book.

If you are looking for a kind of diet that will help you effectively lose, you must try the ketogenic diet. This diet is one of the most effective because it could melt unyielding fats.

Those who have been struggling with weight loss and trying to keep them off but couldn't would understand that the visceral fat are the hardest to lose. But with the ketogenic diet, this is possible.

To get the leaner and fitter physique, this diet teaches the body on how to turn it into usable energy and convert stored fat thereby speeding up weight loss. For first time followers of the Ketogenic diet, it should be noted that carbohydrates found in starchy vegetables, grains, and those in other fruits are not advised to be consumed. Instead, take more of meat, dairy products, seeds, and nuts.

The physiological state that is called ketosis makes it possible for the body to lose more fats. You will learn more about ketosis as you go through the book. This diet also prevents the warning signs of Type II diabetes and delays the onset of Alzheimer's disease. If you are undergoing ketosis, you will notice that you don't feel hungry in between meals and don't crave for sweets and fatty food.

Maintaining a low carbohydrate diet will keep all lifestyle diseases and their complications at bay. This also lessens the risk of stroke and other cardiovascular diseases.

If you want to know more about this diet and the many recipes that you can make, go through the pages of this book and consider this your first step towards welcoming the new you that your future self will thank you for.

Thanks again for purchasing this book. I hope you enjoy it!

Chapter 1 – All about the Ketogenic Diet?

The Ketogenic diet has become popular when it proved effective as means to lose stubborn body fat. It was first designed to control the effects of epilepsy in children. The very principle of this diet is ketosis or the process where the body burns off stored fats.

The body undergoes the state of ketosis the moment glucose from carbohydrates are strictly lessened or totally removed from one's diet. We all know that glucose is the chief fuel of the brain. When you're in ketosis, your brain pushes the pancreas but in such circumstances, the brain rewires and pushes the pancreas to make high amounts of ketone bodies – these are water soluble molecules that breaks down fat in the adipose tissues. The fat converted are absorbed by the brain and becomes the body's energy source.

So, when does ketosis happens? It happens after 2 to 7 days of steady and regular caloric deprivation or what they call the low-carbohydrate consumption. By that time, the human brain is fast burning lipids, converting into free fatty acids, which are processed as an energy fuel. In order to achieve effective weight loss and lifelong health, ketosis should be continued for as long as possible or until you have achieved your desired weight goal. Of course, it would be better if this becomes part of your lifestyle. Note however, that any carbohydrate or sugar intake in the duration of the diet could mean going back to step one. That simply means no cheating on this diet.

Computing your fat intake is simple. All you have to do is get your prescribed number of calories for each day and multiply by 0.70.

The required calories should be between 1,500 to 2,000 calories per day. Divide the result by 9 and you'll get the recommended grams of fat per day. Why divide the result by 9, you might ask? It is because fat contains 9 grams of calories.

Take a look at this sample computation:

1, 500 calories x 0.70 = **1,050** – 9 = **116 grams of fat per day**

The following are food list that you can include in your diet:

Your ketogenic diet should include 70% good, healthy fats such as butter, avocado oil, cocoa butter, coconut butter, coconut oil, olive oil, extra virgin olive oil, fish oil from salmon or tuna among others, sesame oil, lard, walnut oil, palm oil, and flax oil.

Some of the best sources of healthy fats include:

- ✓ Avocadoes – 82.5% fat
- ✓ Bacon – 69.5% fat
- ✓ Butter – 100% fat
- ✓ Cheddar cheese – 74% fat
- ✓ Chicken eggs – 61% fat
- ✓ Coconut flesh/meat – 88% fat
- ✓ Coconut oil – 100% fat
- ✓ Cream cheese – 88.5% fat
- ✓ Sour cream – 88.5% fat
- ✓ Unsweetened dark chocolate – 65% fat
- ✓ Ground beef – 59.5% fat

Fats to avoid:

- x Refined oils such as corn, canola, grape seed oil, rice bran oil, peanut oil, rapeseed oil, soybean oil, cottonseed oil, and sunflower oil.
- x Also, do away with oils that are purified with the use of

hexane solvents, and one that is labeled hydrogenated and partially hydrogenated. These products are linked to cancer producing cells.

It should also be 20% protein. Consuming protein in moderation can help in curbing cravings and will make you feel full for longer hours. Protein is especially beneficial for people who are often working out that helps in sustaining bones and muscles and in burning fats.

This is how you will compute your recommended protein intake per day: Your weight multiplied by 0.6 for the minimum grams of protein per day, and then your weight multiplied by 1.0 if you want to get the maximum grams of protein per day.

Take a look at these figures:

150 pounds x 0.6 = 90 grams (minimum)

150 pounds x 1.0 = 150 grams (maximum)

Some of the best sources of proteins for the ketogenic diet are:

- ✓ Butter
- ✓ Cottage cheese
- ✓ Buttermilk
- ✓ Goat's cheese
- ✓ Feta cheese
- ✓ Cream cheese
- ✓ Sour cream
- ✓ Yogurt
- ✓ Powdered milk
- ✓ Curd
- ✓ Kefir milk
- ✓ Evaporated milk
- ✓ Caught wild such as crab, prawns/shrimps, fish, lobsters,

squid, scallops, mussels, clams, and oysters.
- ✓ Grass-fed such as beef, organ meat, veal, pork, lamb, goat, chicken, turkey, duck, and their eggs.
- ✓ deli meat is allowed in the ketogenic diet provided that they do not contain sugar and starch such as: roasted ham, chicken ham, turkey sausages, corned beef brisket, smoked bacon, salami, and pancetta.
- ✓ Nuts and seeds

Protein to avoid:

- x Filled milk products
- x Condensed milk, frozen custard, ice cream, frozen yogurt, etc.
- x Whey protein
- x artificially flavored and pre-seasoned food

- ✓ 10% net carbohydrates. Acceptable, quality carbs should come from fresh produce, specifically non-starchy and brightly-colored fruits and veggies.

What is Ketosis?

Ketosis is a metabolic state hat the body enters when the ketone levels in the blood reach around 0.5 mmol/L. The by-product of ketosis are ketones. They are a type of acid that accumulate in the blood, which are eliminated in the urine.

Before the word "acid" sends you to a panic mode, let us clarify that the small amount of ketones are harmless. They come as a result of the body's burning and breaking down of fat. They are an indication of the body entering ketosis. However, if ketone levels are too high, it can cause poisoning and will likely lead to a process known as ketoacidosis.

The body does not enter this metabolic state under normal circumstances with your normal diet. It will however, when you restrict your carb consumption. It can also occur when you start fasting for a couple of days. As long as there's sufficiently available carbs from your diet, your body will refuse to enter this metabolic state. In addition, as long as there's remaining stored glycogen in the body or stored form of sugar, the body will not go into ketosis. While sugar is available to provide energy to the cells, the body will refuse to take an alternative fuel supply.

The truth is the body is fine with using glucose as the primary source of fuel. A lot of people never enter the state of ketosis in their lifetime and they still manage to be at an optimum health. Now, you may ask, if you can be at an optimal health without ketosis then what is the purpose of forcing the body to enter ketosis?

What is the purpose of ketosis?

To understand the health purpose of ketosis, a comparison between ketones and sugar will be helpful.

Ketones help the body. And it goes deeper than simply weight loss. It makes the human body work better in the following ways.

-Ketones provide a more efficient source of energy.

-They can help resist aging.

-Ketones can protect the brain and help prevent neurological disorders.

Ketones possesses unique properties that sugar can't. For one thing, ketones are processed and burned in a more efficient manner than sugar ever could. This means ketones are much better as a provider of a more efficient energy source. They also form less reactive oxygen agents. Moreover, ketones have the ability to elevate mitochondrial production and efficiency. This in turn, helps in enhancing the ketone burning cell's ability of producing energy. It also aids in slowing down the process of aging.

According to research, ketones can also act as a neuroprotective antioxidant. It can support in the reversal and prevention of brain damage. At the same time, it triggers the creation of new brain cells and proliferation of connection between brain cells. The process of ketone burning causes a shift of balance in the brain's neurotransmitters, Glutamate and GABA. Excessive neuronal activity can lead to uncontrollable behaviors. This is common among people suffering from neurological disorders such as Parkinson's, autism and epilepsy.

By improving the neurotransmitter balance, ketones assist in protecting the brain from excessive neuronal activity which is helpful for preventing neurological disorders. There are studies that also delve into the way ketosis and ketones can be an effective part of treatment for people suffering from Alzheimer's and certain types of cancer.

Keto Bread Recipes

1. Coconut Nuts Squares

Ingredients:

- 1 cup desiccated coconut
- ½ cup ground almonds
- 4 tablespoons almond butter
- ¼ cup ground walnuts
- ½ cup sunflower seeds
- 3 tablespoons raw honey
- ½ teaspoon sesame oil
- Pinch of sea salt

Directions:

1. Preheat the oven to 350°F. Lightly grease a square baking pan, preferably 8x8 with sesame oil.
2. Meanwhile, put together almonds, coconut, almond butter, walnuts, sunflower seeds, honey and salt in an immersion blender.
3. Process mixture until smooth and no crumbs left. Transfer mixture to the baking pan. Make sure to spread evenly.
4. Place inside the oven and bake for 15 minutes.
5. Allow to cool for a few minutes before slicing into squares. Best consumed when cooled in the fridge.

2. Classic Keto Bread

Ingredients:

- 4 ½ Tbsp. flaxseed meal
- 1/3 tsp. baking soda
- 1/3 tsp. baking powder
- 6 tsp. psyllium powder
- 1/6 tsp. xanthan gum
- 3 tsp. coconut flour
- 3 eggs
- 1/3 cup full fat cream cheese
- 2 Tbsp. coconut oil, melted
- 3 tsp. warm water
- 3 tsp. cider vinegar
- 2 ¼ tsp. stevia
- 1/6 tsp. sea salt

Directions:

1. Preheat the oven to 350 degrees F.
2. Cover baking sheet with baking paper. Set aside.
3. Meanwhile, put together flaxseed meal, baking soda, baking powder, psyllium powder, xanthan gum, and coconut flour in a bowl. Stir well. Set aside.
4. In another bowl, whisk eggs, cream cheese, coconut oil, warm water, cider vinegar, stevia, and salt. Mix well.
5. Gradually pour mix dry ingredients into the bowl of wet ingredients. Mix until smooth.

6. Divide mixture into equal sized rolls. Layer on the baking sheet. Cover with a clean towel. Set aside and allow mixture to rise for 30 minutes to 1 hour.
7. Once risen and the rolls have double their sizes, place inside the oven.
8. Bake for 40 minutes. You'll know when the rolls are cooked once a toothpick inserted comes out clean.
9. Transfer to a cooling rack and let cool for a few minutes before serving.

3. Cardamom Bread

Ingredients:

Dry ingredients

- 4 cups almond flour
- 2¼ teaspoons packet active dry yeast
- 1 teaspoon salt
- 1½ teaspoon maple syrup
- 1¾ cups water, freshly boiled
- 2 tablespoons coconut oil, melted
- Olive oil, for greasing
- ⅛ teaspoon cardamom powder
- ⅛ teaspoon cinnamon powder
- dash of clove powder

Directions:

1. Preheat the oven to 190°C / 375°F for 10 minutes. Combine almond flour, active dry yeast, salt, and maple syrup in a bowl. Create a well in center, and then maple syrup, boiled water, and coconut oil.
2. Mix all ingredients until dough comes together. On a floured surface, turn out the dough and create a depression at the center.
3. Add in cardamom powder, cinnamon powder, and garlic powder. Knead for 10 minutes, or until the dough is elastic. If the dough is sticky, add more flour.
4. Grease the same bowl with oil. Put the dough. Cover with saran wrap and the dough rise for 1 hour, or until it becomes double the size.
5. Grease the bread loaf pans.

6. Once rise, punch dough down. Turn out on the floured surface. Divide in half.
7. Form dough into a loaf, tucking, and stretching the edges.
8. Place in the loaf pans. Cover with saran wrap and let it rise for 20 minutes.
9. Place loaf pans in the middle rack and bake for 40 minutes. You'll know that the loaves are cooked once they turn golden brown in color.
10. Place on cooling racks. Once cooled, remove loaves from the pan. Slice and serve.

4. Keto Bacon and Cheese Bread

Ingredients:

- 1 ½ cups almond flour
- ½ cup bacon, diced
- 1 tbsp. baking powder
- 2 eggs
- 4 tbsp. butter, melted
- 1/3 cup sour cream
- 1 cup cheddar cheese, grated

Directions:

1. Preheat the oven to 300°F. Lightly grease a loaf tin and line with parchment paper.
2. Meanwhile, in a nonstick skillet, cook the bacon pieces until crisp. Set aside.
3. Combine almond flour and baking powder. Mix well.
4. In another bowl, put together sour cream and eggs. Whisk until smooth.
5. Pour egg mixture into the flour mixture. Mix well.
6. Add melted butter. Fold bacon and cheese into the batter. Mix.
7. Transfer to the loaf tin. Place inside the oven and bake for 45 minutes. You'll know when the rolls are cooked once a toothpick inserted comes out clean.
8. Allow to cool for a few minutes before slicing. Serve.

5. Cheese and Garlic Bread

Ingredients:

- ½ tsp. cream of tartar
- 4 eggs, separate yolks from the whites
- ¼ tsp. garlic powder
- 2 oz. cream cheese
- 1 tsp. Italian seasoning
- ½ tsp. sea salt

Directions:

1. Preheat the oven to 300°F. Line a baking sheet with parchment paper.
2. Meanwhile, put together cream of tartar and egg whites in a bowl. Mix well until stiff peaks form.
3. In another bowl, place cream cheese and beat. Add in egg yolks. Mix continuously until the mixture is smooth.
4. Continue to mix until smooth. Add in garlic powder, Italian seasoning, and salt.
5. Fold in egg whites into the yolk mixture. Continue to fold to until the mixture is firm and foamy.
6. Place batter onto the baking sheets. Spread into 4-inch rounds about 4-inch and ¾ inch high.
7. Place inside the oven and bake for 30 minutes until golden brown in color. Let cool for a few minutes before removing from the baking sheet. Serve.

6. Blueberry Loaf

Ingredients:

- ½ cup almond flour
- 2 tbsp. baking powder
- ½ cup blueberries
- ½ tsp. salt
- ½ cup almond butter, melted
- ¼ cup ghee, melted
- ½ cup almond milk, unsweetened
- 5 eggs, beaten

Directions:

1. Preheat the oven to 350°F. Grease a loaf tin and line with parchment paper.
2. Mix together almond flour, baking powder, and salt in a bowl. Stir in almond butter and ghee. Mix until all ingredients are combined well.
3. Whisk the eggs and milk together before adding to the bowl. Mix well,
4. Scatter blueberries into the batter and pour into the loaf tin.
5. Place inside the oven and bake for 45 minutes. You'll know when the rolls are cooked once a toothpick inserted comes out clean.
6. Allow the bread to cool completely before removing from the tin and slicing.

7. 10-Minute Bread

Ingredients:

- 1 large egg
- 3 tbsp. almond flour
- ½ tsp. baking powder
- 1 tbsp. butter, melted

Directions:

1. Preheat the oven to 325 degrees F.
2. Meanwhile, combine almond flour, egg, baking powder, and butter in a ramekin. Mix well until all ingredients are well-incorporated.
3. Place inside the microwave oven and heat for 90 seconds.
4. Transfer to the oven and bake for 10 minutes. Serve.

11. Keto Loaf

Ingredients:

- 2 cups almond flour
- 1 teaspoon baking powder
- ½ teaspoon xanthan gum (optional)
- 7 eggs at room temperature
- ½ cup melted butter
- 2 tablespoons olive or coconut oil, melted
- A dash of salt

Directions:

1. Preheat the oven to 325F.
2. Lightly grease a loaf pan with oil. Line with baking paper. Set aside.
3. Meanwhile, put together baking powder, almond flour, xanthan gum, and salt in a bowl. Set aside.
4. In a separate bowl, beat all the eggs. Add in oil and butter. Whisk well until pale in color.
5. Fold in the almond mixture in two or three additions. Stir until well combined. Do not over mix or the bread would be too hard.
6. Pour in the prepared loaf pan. Bake in the middle or in the top shelf for 40 minutes. You'll know when the rolls are cooked once a toothpick inserted comes out clean.
7. Let bread cool before slicing and serving.

12. Sesame Seed Loaf

Ingredients:

- 2 tablespoons chia seeds
- 1 tablespoon sesame seeds
- 1 teaspoon baking powder
- 2 cups almond flour
- 7 eggs
- ½ cup butter, melted
- 2 tablespoons flaxseed oil
- Pinch of salt

Directions:

1. Preheat the oven to 350F. Grease a loaf pan with butter.
2. Meanwhile, put together chia seeds, almond flour, baking powder, and salt. Set aside.
3. In another bowl, beat the eggs until frothy. Pour oil and stir in butter. Mix well.
4. Gradually add the dry ingredients into the wet ingredients.
5. Pour egg mixture into the flour mixture.
6. Place inside the oven and bake for 15 minutes. Scatter sesame seeds on top of the loaf.
7. Bake for another 15 minutes. Let cool before slicing and serving.

13. Blueberry with Icing Keto Bread

Ingredients:

- 6 eggs
- 10 tbsp. coconut flour
- 2/3 cup Monkfruit sweetener
- 9 tbsp. butter, melted
- ¾ cup blueberries
- 1 ½ tsp. baking powder
- 2 tbsp. sour cream
- 2 tbsp. heavy whipping cream
- 1 ½ tsp. vanilla
- ½ tsp. salt
- ½ tsp. cinnamon

For the Icing

- 1 tbsp. heavy whipping cream
- 2 tbsp. Monkfruit sweetener
- 1 tsp. butter, melted
- ¼ tsp. lemon zest
- 1/8 tsp. vanilla

Directions:

1. Preheat the oven to 350°F. Line a loaf tin with parchment paper.
2. Meanwhile, put together eggs, coconut flour, Monkfruit sweetener, butter, blueberries, baking powder, sour cream, whipping cream, vanilla, salt, and cinnamon. Mix well.

3. Place just the right amount of batter into the loaf tin. Top with blueberries.
4. Repeat the method until all the batter and blueberries are used up.
5. Place inside the oven and bake for 1 hour and 5 minutes. You'll know when the rolls are cooked once a toothpick inserted comes out clean.
6. Let cool for 5 minutes. While the bread is cooling, put together heavy whipping cream, Monkfruit sweetener, butter, lemon zest, and vanilla. Whisk until smooth.
7. Slice the bread and drizzle in icing on top. Serve.

Recipe #2 - Coriander Bread

Ingredients:

Dry ingredients

- 4 cups almond flour
- 2¼ teaspoons active dry yeast
- 2/3 cup Monkfruit sweetener
- 1 teaspoon kosher salt

Wet ingredients

- 1¾ cups freshly boiled water
- 2 tablespoons coconut oil, melted
- 1 teaspoon vinegar

Aromatics

- ⅛ cup fresh coriander, mince
- 1 teaspoons coriander seeds, divided

Directions:

1. Combine dry ingredients into large mixing bowl. Make well in center. Pour in wet ingredients.
2. With a wooden spoon, gradually mix dry and wet ingredients until dough comes together. Turn out dough on floured surface; make depression in middle. Add in fresh coriander; knead until elastic, about 7 to 10 minutes Add flour if dough is too sticky.

3. Lightly grease (same) bowl with oil. Place dough in. Cover bowl with saran wrap. Let dough rise in a warm place for 1 to 1½ hours, or until double in size.
4. Lightly grease bread loaf pans.
5. Punch dough down; turn out on floured surface. Divide in half. Form dough into rough loaf, stretching, and tucking in edges underneath; place in prepared loaf pans. Let dough rise for 20 minutes, covered loosely with saran wrap.
6. Preheat oven to 190°C / 375°F for 10 minutes.
7. Add equal amounts of coriander seeds on top of dough. Place pans on middle rack of oven. Bake for 35 minutes, or until bread top is golden brown.
8. Remove pans from oven and set on cooling racks. When pan is cool enough to handle, remove loaves. Allow bread to cool further before slicing.

14. Almond Loaf

Ingredients:

- 1/3 cup flaxseed meal
- 1 ½ cup almond flour
- 2 teaspoons baking powder
- ¼ cup almond milk, unsweetened
- 2 tablespoons coconut oil, melted
- 4 eggs
- Pinch of salt
- Coconut oil, for greasing

Direction:

1. Preheat the oven to 350F.
2. Grease loaf pan with coconut oil.
3. Put together flaxseed meal, almond flour, baking powder, almond milk, coconut oil, eggs, and salt in a bowl. Mix until a smooth dough forms.
4. Press the dough on the loaf pan. Leave for 10 minutes.
5. Place inside the oven and bake for 50 minutes. You'll know when the rolls are cooked once a toothpick inserted comes out clean.
6. Allow the bread to cool for 15 minutes before slicing and serving.

15. Yolk-less Keto Bread

Ingredients:

- 1 cup almond flour
- 2 teaspoons baking powder
- ¼ cup coconut flour
- Pinch of salt
- 12 egg whites
- ¼ teaspoon cream of tartar
- 1/3 cup butter, melted

Directions:

1. Preheat the oven to 325F. Grease the pan and line with parchment paper
2. Meanwhile, in a bowl, put together all ingredients except for cream of tartar and egg whites. Stir until a soft dough forms.
3. In another bowl, beat eggs and cream of tartar into the mixture until stiff peaks form.
4. Gradually fold egg whites into the dough. Add more eggs if the dough is a bit hard.
5. Place inside the oven and bake for 30 minutes. Cover the top with aluminum foil and bake for another 45 minutes.
6. Allow to cool before peeling off parchment paper and slicing.

16. Cheesy Peperoni Loaf

Ingredients:

- ½ cup coconut flour
- 1 tsp. baking powder
- ½ spring onion, finely chopped
- 1 cup cheddar cheese, grated
- 1 stick of pepperoni, sliced thinly
- Dash of chili
- pinch of salt
- Pinch of pepper
- 2 tbsp. pumpkin seeds
- 8 eggs
- ½ cup butter, softened

Directions:

1. Preheat the oven to 350°. Grease a loaf pan with butter.
2. Meanwhile, put together coconut flour, baking powder, salt, pepper, butter, and chili in a bowl. Mix until all ingredients come together.
3. Beat eggs one at a time into the bowl whilst stirring.
4. Add in cheese and spring onions.
5. Transfer mixture into the loaf tin. Top with pumpkin seeds, pepperoni, and cheese.
6. Place inside the oven and bake for 15 minutes or until golden brown. Let cool before serving.

17. Garlic and Cauliflower Bread

Ingredients:

- 3 tablespoons of garlic, minced
- 1 teaspoon dried oregano
- 3 tablespoons of olive oil
- 6 large eggs
- 6 tablespoons of coconut oil, divided
- 2 tablespoons baking powder
- 1 ¼ cup almond flour
- 2 large heads cauliflower, grind in a food processor
- 1 teaspoon salt
- Pinch of white pepper
- Pinch of cream of tartar

Directions:

1. Heat half the oil in a pan. Saute garlic until browned all over. Set aside.
2. In the same pan, saute cauliflower until cooked.
3. Transfer cauliflower in a clean towel. Let dry. Cook in batches if necessary. Set aside.
4. In a different bowl, beat the eggs. Add in the remaining oil, almond flour, baking powder, salt, and pepper in the egg yolk. Whisk well. Fold in cauliflower rice. Set aside.
5. Meanwhile, beat egg whites until frothy using an electric mixer. Add in cream of tartar. Continue beating.
6. Add in one third of egg whites to the egg yolk mixture. Beat well.
7. Fold in the rest of the egg whites into the yolk mixture. No need to mix.
8. Pour into the pan. Scatter garlic all over.

9. Place inside the oven and bake for 50 minutes. You'll know when the rolls are cooked once a toothpick inserted comes out clean.
10. Check after 30 minutes of baking. Cover top with aluminum foil. Check every five minutes.
11. Allow to cool before slicing.

18. Macadamia Bread

Ingredients:

- ½ tsp. baking powder
- 1 cup coconut flour, sifted
- ½ tbsp. psyllium husk powder
- ¼ tsp. salt
- 2 cup macadamia butter
- ½ tsp. Erythritol sweetener
- 2 eggs
- 1 egg white

Directions:

1. Preheat the oven to 350°. Line a baking sheet with parchment paper.
2. Combine baking powder, coconut flour, psyllium husk powder, and salt in a bowl. Mix well.
3. In another bowl, beat eggs, sweetener, and macadamia butter.
4. Put together the four and egg mixture. Add flour if the mixture is watery.
5. Divide dough into disks, and then transfer to a Place the dough disks onto the baking sheet.
6. Place inside the oven and bake for 30 minutes. You'll know when the rolls are cooked once a toothpick inserted comes out clean.
7. Allow the bread to cool for 15 minutes before slicing and serving.

19. Almond Bread

Ingredients:

- ½ cup Stevia sweetener
- ½ cup heavy cream
- ½ cup butter
- 2 egg
- 1 tsp. baking powder
- 2 ¼ cups almond flour
- ¼ tsp. ginger powder
- 2 tbsp. ground flaxseed
- ½ tsp. xanthan gum
- ¼ tsp. ground star anise

Directions:

1. Preheat the oven to 350°F. Line loaf tin with parchment paper.
2. Melt the butter in a pan. Add in stevia and heavy cream. Mix well until the sugar dissolves.
3. Remove from heat. Set aside for a few minutes to cool.
4. In a bowl, put together baking powder, almond flour, ginger powder, ground flaxseed, xanthan gum, and ground star anise.
5. Stir in eggs and the butter mixture. Stir well.
6. Pour batter into the tin. Place inside the oven and bake for 45 minutes, covered.
7. Allow the bread to cool for 15 minutes before slicing and serving.

20. Cinnamon Bread

Ingredients:

- 2 teaspoons baking powder
- 1 cup almond flour
- 1/3 cup flaxseed meal
- ½ cup coconut flour
- Pinch of salt
- 4 eggs
- 2 tablespoons coconut oil, melted
- ¼ cup almond milk, unsweetened
- ¼ cup butter, softened
- 1 teaspoon cinnamon
- 2 tablespoons coconut flour, for dusting

Direction:

1. Preheat the oven to 350 degrees F.
2. Grease a loaf pan with butter. Dust the sides of the pan with coconut flour.
3. Put together baking powder, almond flour, flaxseed meal, coconut flour, salt, eggs, coconut oil, and almond milk in a bowl. Mix well until it forms a dough.
4. Press dough into the pan.
5. Meanwhile, in a different bowl, mix cinnamon and butter. Pour mixture on the pan.
6. Spread mixture in a swirling motion. Pour the other half on top of the cinnamon-butter mix.
7. Place inside the oven and bake for 30 minutes.
8. You'll know when the rolls are cooked once a toothpick inserted comes out clean.

9. Allow the bread to cool for 15 minutes before slicing and serving.

21. Coconut Loaf

Ingredients:

- 2 cups coconut flour
- 2 teaspoon baking powder
- ½ teaspoon xanthan gum
- Pinch of salt
- 4 egg yolks
- 7 egg whites
- ½ cup butter, melted
- 2 tablespoons coconut oil, melted

Direction:

1. Line a loaf pan with baking paper. Set aside.
2. In a bowl, put together coconut flour, baking powder, xanthan gum, and salt. Mix well.
3. In another bowl, beat the egg whites, butter, and coconut oil.
4. Pour flour mixture into the egg mixture. Beat until soft peaks form.
5. Spoon just the right amount of egg white to the egg yolk. Mix well.
6. Pour into the loaf pan. Place in the middle part of the oven and bake for 30 minutes.
7. You'll know when the rolls are cooked once a toothpick inserted comes out clean.
8. Allow the bread to cool for 15 minutes before slicing and serving.

22. Vegetables and Seeds Loaf

Ingredients:

- 1/3 cup coconut flour
- 1 cup almond flour
- 2 tbsp. psyllium husk powder
- 2 tsp. baking powder
- 2 tsp. pink Himalayan salt
- 1 tbsp. paprika, smoked
- 2 tsp. cumin, ground
- 1 zucchini, grated
- 1 cup pumpkin, grated
- 1 carrot, grated
- ½ cup sunflower
- ½ cup flaxseeds
- ½ cup sesame seeds
- ¼ cup coconut oil or ghee
- 4 large eggs

Directions:

1. Preheat the oven to 340°F. Line a loaf tin with parchment paper.
2. In a large bowl, mix the almond and coconut flours, salt, spices, baking powder, mixed seeds, and psyllium husk powder until they're well-combined.
3. In a separate bowl, combine grated zucchini, pumpkin, and carrot, eggs, and coconut oil.
4. Pour flour mixture into the vegetable mix. Stir well until all ingredients are well-incorporated.

5. Transfer to the loaf tin. Sprinkle sunflower, flaxseeds, and sesame seeds on top.
6. Place inside the oven and bake for 50 minutes.
7. You'll know when the rolls are cooked once a toothpick inserted comes out clean.
8. Allow the bread to cool for 15 minutes before slicing and serving.

23. Black Sesame Seed Bread

Ingredients:

- 1 teaspoon baking powder
- 2 cups hemp seed flour
- ½ teaspoon xanthan gum
- Pinch of salt
- 1 tablespoon black sesame seeds
- 7 eggs
- ½ cup olive oil
- 2 tablespoons butter, melted

Directions:

1. Preheat the oven to 175C. Grease loaf pan with oil. Line with parchment paper. Set aside.
2. Put together baking powder, hemp seed flour, xanthan gum, and salt in a bowl. Mix.
3. In another bowl, beat the eggs. Add in butter and oil. Stir well.
4. Pour batter into the loaf pan.
5. Place inside the oven and bake for 20 minutes. Scatter sesame seeds on top. Cook for another 15 minutes.
6. You'll know when the rolls are cooked once a toothpick inserted comes out clean.
7. Allow the bread to cool for 15 minutes before slicing and serving.

24. Onion Bread

Ingredients:

- 1 teaspoon baking powder
- 2 cups hemp seed flour
- ½ teaspoon xanthan gum
- Pinch of salt
- 1 large onion, sliced thinly
- 7 eggs
- ½ cup olive oil
- 2 tablespoons butter, melted

Directions:

1. Preheat the oven to 175C. Grease loaf pan with oil. Line with parchment paper. Set aside.
2. Put together baking powder, hemp seed flour, xanthan gum, and salt in a bowl. Mix.
3. In another bowl, beat the eggs. Add in butter and oil. Stir well.
4. Pour batter into the loaf pan.
5. Meanwhile, cook onions in a nonstick skillet for 10 minutes, or until it caramelizes.
6. Place inside the oven and bake for 20 minutes. Scatter cooked onions on top. Cook for another 15 minutes.
7. You'll know when the rolls are cooked once a toothpick inserted comes out clean.
8. Allow the bread to cool for 15 minutes before slicing and serving.

25. Zucchini and Pecans Bread

Ingredients:

- 8 eggs
- 1 tsp. baking soda
- 1 ½ tsp. baking powder
- 1 tbsp. coconut flour
- 1 cup almond flour
- 2/3 cup zucchini, grated
- ½ cup Monkfruit
- ¼ cup pecans, chopped
- 1 tsp. cinnamon
- ½ tsp salt
- 1 tsp. vanilla extract
- 3 tbsp. sour cream
- 1/3 cup butter, melted

Directions:

1. Preheat the oven to 350°F. Grease a loaf tin with oil. Line with parchment paper.
2. Beat the eggs until foamy.
3. Add in baking soda, baking powder, coconut flour, almond flour, zucchini, monkfruit, pecans, cinnamon, and salt. Mix until all ingredients are well-incorporated.
4. Transfer to the loaf tin. Sprinkle pecans on top.
5. Place inside the oven and bake for 35 minutes. O the 15th minute mark, cover with parchment paper.
6. You'll know when the rolls are cooked once a toothpick inserted comes out clean.
7. Allow the bread to cool for 15 minutes before slicing and serving.

Chapter 3: Muffins, Bagels, and Buns

26. Fruity Muffins

Ingredients:

- 2 cups almond flour
- 3 teaspoons baking powder
- ½ teaspoon salt
- 2 eggs
- ½ cup agave
- ¼ cup oil
- ¾ cup sour soy milk
- 1 ½ cups keto-approved frozen fruits of choice

Directions:

1. Preheat the oven to 350 degrees F.
2. Combine flour, baking powder, and salt in a bowl. Add egg, sweetener, oil, sour milk, and fruit. Mix well.
3. Scoop into muffin tins.
4. Place inside the oven and bake for 30 minutes.
5. Allow the bread to cool for 15 minutes before serving.

27. Zucchini Muffins

Ingredients:

- 2 cups zucchini, grated
- ¾ cup almond flour
- 1 teaspoon baking powder
- Pinch of salt
- Pinch of pepper
- ½ cup cream cheese, softened
- ½ cup butter, softened
- 6 eggs

Directions:

1. Preheat the oven to 350 degrees F.
2. Put together almond flour and baking powder. Set aside.
3. Meanwhile, combine butter, zucchini, salt, and pepper. Mix well.
4. Pour beaten eggs into the mixture. Fold in cream cheese.
5. Pour batter into the muffin tray. Place inside the oven and bake for 20 minutes. Serve.

28. Herbed and Cheese Bun

Ingredients:

- 1 cup coconut flour
- 1 teaspoon baking powder
- 1 teaspoon garlic, minced
- ¼ cup onion, minced
- 5/8 cups cream cheese
- Pinch of salt
- Pinch of pepper
- ¼ cup butter
- 1 egg
- Sesame seeds, for topping

Direction:

1. Preheat the oven to 350F. Grease a muffin pan with oil.
2. Combine butter and cream cheese in a bowl. Using an electric mixer, beat the mixture. Add in cream and egg once again.
3. Stir in garlic, onion, salt, and pepper. Mix well.
4. In a separate bowl, mix the flour and baking powder. Pour into the cheese mixture.
5. Pour just the right amount of batter into the muffin pan. Sprinkle sesame seeds on top.
6. Place inside the oven and bake for 20 minutes.
7. Allow bread to cool for 15 minutes before serving.

29. Everything Cheese Bagels

Ingredients:

- 2 eggs
- 2 tbsp. everything bagel seasoning
- 1 cup mozzarella cheese
- ½ cup parmesan cheese

Directions:

1. Preheat the oven to 375°F. Lightly grease a donut pan.
2. Meanwhile, put together eggs, everything bagel seasoning, mozzarella cheese, and parmesan cheese in a bowl. Mix until all ingredients come together.
3. Press just the right amount of mixture into the donut pan. Sperinkle bagel seasoning on top of each.
4. Place inside the ovben and bake for 20 minuyte, or until the cheese melts.
5. Let cool before serving.

30. Cauliflower and Cheese Muffin

Ingredients:

- 2 cups cauliflower rice, grated
- ¾ cup almond flour
- 1 teaspoon baking powder
- Pinch of salt
- Pinch of pepper
- 1 cup cream cheese
- ½ cup mozzarella cheese
- ½ cup butter, softened
- 6 eggs

Directions:

1. Preheat the oven to 350 degrees F.
2. Put together almond flour and baking powder. Set aside.
3. Meanwhile, combine butter, cauliflower rice, salt, and pepper. Mix well.
4. Pour beaten eggs into the mixture. Fold in cream cheese and mozarella cheese.
5. Pour batter into the muffin tray. Place inside the oven and bake for 20 minutes. Serve.

31. Carrots Cashew Muffins

Ingredients:

- 4 eggs
- 1½ cups almond flour
- 2 teaspoons baking soda
- 4 carrots, processed
- ½ cup maple syrup
- ¼ cup coconut oil
- ¼ cup cashew nuts, chopped
- 1 teaspoon vanilla extract

Directions:

1. Preheat the oven to 375°F. Line muffin tins with paper liners.
2. Put together carrots, eggs, almond flour, baking soda, maple syrup, coconut oil, cashew nuts, and vanilla extract in a bowl. mix.
3. Spoon equal amounts of batter into the muffin depressions. Place inside the oven and bake for 20 minutes.
4. You'll know when the rolls are cooked once a toothpick inserted comes out clean.
5. Let cool before removing from tins. Serve.

32. Zucchini and Cheese Muffins

Ingredients:

- 2 cups zucchini, grated
- ½ cup butter, softened
- ¾ cup almond flour
- 1 teaspoon baking powder
- Pinch of salt
- Pinch of pepper
- 6 eggs
- ½ cup cream cheese, softened
- 1 cup cheddar cheese

Directions:

1. Preheat the oven to 350 degrees F.
2. Put together almond flour and baking powder. Set aside.
3. Meanwhile, combine butter, zucchini, salt, and pepper. Mix well.
4. Pour beaten eggs into the mixture. Fold in cheddar cheese.
5. Pour batter into the muffin tray. Place inside the oven and bake for 20 minutes. Serve.

33. Caraway and Cheese Bagels

Ingredients:

- 1 large egg
- 1 cup cream cheese
- 1 cup almond flour
- 1 ½ tsp. baking powder
- ½ tbsp. cocoa powder
- 1 ½ cups mozzarella, shredded
- 1 tsp. caraway seeds
- 1 tsp. yacon syrup

Directions:

1. Preheat the oven to 325°F. Line a baking sheet with parchment paper.
2. Beast the egg in a bowl. Set aside.
3. In another bowl, mix almond flour, baking powder, cocoa powder, caraway seeds, and yacon syrup until all ingredients come together.
4. Meanwhile, place mozarella and cream cheese in a microwave oven. Heat for 1 minute. Stir every 30 seconds.
5. Pour cheese mixture on the egg, and then to the flour mixture. Mix until a dough forms.
6. Shape dough into bagels. Place on the baking sheet. Place inside the oven and bake for 15 minutes or until golden brown.
7. Allow to cool before serving.

34. Spicy and Cheesy Jalapeno Bagels

Ingredients:

- 3 jalapenos, thinly sliced
- 1 cup almond flour
- 1 tsp. baking powder
- 1 cup cream cheese
- 2 cups mozzarella, grated
- 1 cup cheddar, grated
- 2 eggs

Directions:

1. Preheat the oven to 400°F. Lightly grease a bagel pan with oil.
2. Put together almond flour and baking powder in a bowl. Beat the eggs and add in jalapenos. Mix well.
3. Meanwhile, place mozarella and cream cheese in a microwave oven. Heat for 1 minute. Stir every 30 seconds.
4. Mix until a dough forms.
5. Shape dough into bagels. Place on the baking sheet. Place inside the oven and bake for 25 minutes or until golden brown.
6. Allow to cool before serving.

35. Microwaveable Bun

Ingredients:

- 1 egg
- 3 tbsp. almond flour
- ½ tsp. baking powder
- 1 ½ tbsp. olive oil

Directions:

1. Put together almond flour and baking powder in a bowl. Mix well, making sure that all lumps are removed and the mixture smooth.
2. Beat in egg and oil. Whisk until blended well.
3. Microwave bread for 90 seconds. Serve with butter or peanut butter.

36. Keto Hamburger

Ingredients:

- 3 egg whites
- 1 teaspoon apple cider vinegar
- 1 whole egg
- 1 cup boiling water
- 3/4 cup hemp seed flour
- 1/4 cup coconut flour
- 1 teaspoon baking powder
- 1/4 cup flaxseed meal
- 1 teaspoon xanthan gum
- 1 teaspoon garlic powder
- Sesame seeds, for toppings

Directions:

1. Preheat the oven to 350F.
2. Put together hemp seed flour, coconut flour, baking powder, flaxseed meal, xanthan gum, and garlic powder in a bowl. Mix well.
3. In a separate bowl, add in whole eggs, egg whites, and apple cider vinegar. Mix well. Pour mixture into the flour mix.
4. Meanwhile, boil water in a sauce pan. Pour the batter. Mix until a dough-like consistency is achieved.
5. Shape each into a ball. Layer on the baking sheet. Scatter sesame seeds on top.
6. Place inside the oven and bake for 50 minutes.
7. You'll know when the rolls are cooked once a toothpick inserted comes out clean.
8. Let cool before slicing. Serve.

37. Pure Almond Flour Bun

Ingredients:

- 3 egg whites
- 1 teaspoon apple cider vinegar
- 1 whole egg
- 1 cup boiling water
- 1/2 cup almond flour
- 1 teaspoon baking powder
- 1/4 cup flaxseed meal
- 1 teaspoon xanthan gum
- Sesame seeds, for toppings

Directions:

1. Preheat the oven to 350F.
2. Put together almond flour, baking powder, flaxseed meal, and xanthan gum in a bowl. Mix well.
3. In a separate bowl, add in whole eggs, egg whites, and apple cider vinegar. Mix well. Pour mixture into the flour mix.
4. Meanwhile, boil water in a sauce pan. Pour the batter. Mix until a dough-like consistency is achieved.
5. Shape each into a ball. Layer on the baking sheet. Scatter sesame seeds on top.
6. Place inside the oven and bake for 50 minutes.
7. You'll know when the rolls are cooked once a toothpick inserted comes out clean.
8. Let cool before slicing. Serve.

38. Cauliflower Bun

Ingredients

- 2 heads cauliflower
- ½ cup Parmesan cheese, shredded
- 2 eggs
- 4 tablespoons of coconut flour
- ½ teaspoon baking powder
- Pinch of salt
- Pinch of pepper
- Dash of onion powder
- Dash of garlic powder
- ½ teaspoon sesame seeds

Directions:

1. Chop the cauliflower. Place it in the food processor and grind into fine crumbs. Set aside 3 cups. Dry the cauliflower rice. Use the technique discussed in Garlic and Cauliflower Loaf in Chapter 3.
2. Place the dry cauliflower and the rest of the dry ingredients in a bowl. Break in the two eggs and mix by hand or by spatula until a soft dough forms.
3. Divide the dough into 6 portions. Roll them into a ball or any desired shape.
4. Arrange on a greased baking sheet. Bake in a 200C (400F) preheated oven for 20 to 25 minutes. Serve hot

39. Cranberries with Walnuts Muffins

Ingredients:

- 1 serving flax egg
- 1¾ cup all-purpose flour
- 1⅛ cups walnut milk
- ½ cup fresh cranberries, rinsed, drained
- ¼ cup coconut oil
- ¼ cup shelled walnuts, roughly chopped
- 3 tablespoons palm sugar, crumbled
- 2 teaspoons baking powder
- ½ teaspoon kosher salt

Directions:

1. Preheat oven to 375°F or 190°C. Place paper liners into muffin tins. Combine ingredients in large mixing bowl. Do not over mix.
2. Spoon equal portions of batter into 10 or 11 paper lined muffin depressions. Bake for 20 to 22 minutes, or until toothpick comes out clean.
3. Remove from oven immediately. Cool slightly before removing muffins from tins. Place muffins on cake rack to cool further. Serve.

40. Spinach and Feta Muffin

Ingredients:

- 2 tbsp. feta, grated
- 1 tbsp. spinach
- Dash of baking soda
- Pinch of salt
- 1 egg
- 2 tsp. coconut flour

Directions:

1. Preheat the oven to 400 degrees F.
2. Grease a ramekin dish with coconut oil.
3. Put together feta, spinach, baking soda, salt, egg, and coconut flour in a bowl.
4. Place inside the oven and bake for 45 minutes.
5. Let cool before removing from the ramekin dish. Serve.

41. All Herbed Muffins

Ingredients:

- 1 cup almond flour, blanched
- 3 tbsp. coconut flour
- 2 tsp. baking powder
- 1 tsp. Erythritol sweetener
- ½ tsp. fresh thyme
- ¼ tsp. xanthan gum
- ¾ tsp. salt
- ¼ tsp. garlic powder
- ½ cup sharp cheddar, grated
- 2 eggs
- 1/3 cup unsweetened almond milk
- 6 tbsp. butter, melted

Directions:

1. Preheat the oven to 375°F. Grease muffin tins.
2. Meanwhile, put together almond flour, coconut flour, baking powder, Erythritol sweetener, thyme, xanthan gum, salt, garlic powder, and cheddar in a bowl.
3. In a separate bowl, add in eggs, almond milk, and butter. Whisk well.
4. Pour egg mixture into the flour mixture.
5. Pour batter into each muffin tin.
6. Place inside the oven and bake for 25 minutes.
7. You'll know when the rolls are cooked once a toothpick inserted comes out clean.
8. Let cool before removing from tins. Serve.

42. Cauliflower and Herbed Bun

Ingredients:

- 2 cauliflower heads, chopped, grounded into crumbs using a processor
- ½ teaspoon baking powder
- 4 tablespoons coconut flour
- Dash of garlic powder
- Dash of onion powder
- ½ cup Parmesan cheese, shredded
- Pinch of salt
- Pinch of pepper
- 2 eggs
- ½ teaspoon sesame seeds

Directions:

1. Preheat the oven to 40 degrees F. Lightly grease baking sheet.
2. Place cauliflower crumbs in a bowl. Add in a baking powder, coconut flour, garlic powder, onion powder, Parmesan cheese, salt, and pepper. Mix well.
3. In another bowl, beat the eggs. Whisk until soft dough forms. Add more flour if the dough has more water.
4. Roll dough into balls. Place inside the oven and bake for 25 minutes. Serve hot.

43. Three-Chesses Bagel

Ingredients:

- ½ cup cheddar cheese
- 1 ½ cups of almond flour
- 2 teaspoons xanthan gum
- 3 cups mozzarella cheese
- 4 tablespoons cream cheese
- 2 eggs

Direction:

1. Preheat the oven to 400 degrees F.
2. In a microwavable bowl, put mozzarella cheese and cream cheese.
3. In another bowl, put together xanthan gum and flour.
4. Place chesses inside the microwave oven and heat for 1 minute. Stir and then put back to the microwave to heat for 30 seconds.
5. Gradually add in flour mixture. Mix well.
6. In a separate bowl, beat the eggs and pour over the flour mix. Knead until elastic.
7. Shape into a ball. Layer on the baking sheet. Flatten ball and create a hole in the center.
8. Scatter cheese on top with rosemary and oregano.
9. Place inside the oven and bake for 18 minutes. Serve.

Variety:

- **Sesame cheese bagel.** Sprinkle sesame seeds on top instead of cheese.

44. Chicken and Bacon Muffins

Ingredients:

- ½ cup coconut milk
- 1 chicken breast, diced
- 2 bacon slices, diced
- 2 tbsp. thyme, chopped
- 1 carrot, grated
- Pinch of salt
- Pinch of pepper
- 1 tbsp. coconut oil
- 8 eggs

Directions:

1. Preheat the oven to 350°F.
2. In a pan, heat the coconut oil. Cook bacon and chicken until browned all over.
3. Transfer cooked meat to a bowl.
4. Saute carrots and thyme. Season with salt and pepper. Cook until tender.
5. In a separate bowl, beat the eggs and coconut cream and eggs. Mix well. Pour into the chicken mixture.
6. Spoon into muffin tins. Place inside the oven and bake for 30 minutes. Let cool before serving.

45. Pizza-Style Bagel

Ingredients:

- ½ cup cheddar cheese
- 1 ½ cups of almond flour
- 2 teaspoons xanthan gum
- 3 cups mozzarella cheese
- ½ cup red and green bell pepper
- ½ cup ground beef
- 4 tablespoons cream cheese
- 2 eggs

Direction:

1. Preheat the oven to 400 degrees F.
2. In a microwavable bowl, put mozzarella cheese and cream cheese.
3. In another bowl, put together xanthan gum and flour.
4. Place chesses inside the microwave oven and heat for 1 minute. Stir and then put back to the microwave to heat for 30 seconds.
5. Gradually add in flour mixture. Mix well.
6. In a separate bowl, beat the eggs and pour over the flour mix. Knead until elastic.
7. Shape into a ball. Layer on the baking sheet. Flatten ball and press the dough to make a crust. Spread keto-approved tomato sauce.
8. Scatter ground beef, bell peppers, and cheeses on top.
9. Place inside the oven and bake for 18 minutes. Serve

46. Corn with Raspberries Muffins

Ingredients:

- 1 serving flax egg
- 1 ¾ cup whole wheat pastry flour
- 1 ⅛ cup coconut milk
- ½ cup fresh raspberries, rinsed, drained
- ¼ cup coconut oil
- ¼ cup canned, whole corn kernels, rinsed, drained
- 3 tablespoons palm sugar
- 2 teaspoons baking powder
- ½ teaspoon kosher salt

Directions:

1. Preheat oven to 375°F or 190°C. Place paper liners into muffin tins. Combine ingredients in large mixing bowl. Do not over mix.
2. Spoon equal portions of batter into 10 or 11 paper lined muffin depressions. Bake for 20 to 22 minutes, or until toothpick comes out clean. Remove from oven immediately.
3. Cool slightly before removing muffins from tins. Place muffins on cake rack to cool further. Serve.

47. Choco Cocoa Muffins

Ingredients:

- 3 oz. butter, unsalted, melted
- 1 cup almond flour
- 2/3 cup heavy cream
- ½ cup Erythritol sweetener
- ½ cup cocoa powder, unsweetened
- ½ cup chocolate chips, sugar-free
- 1 ½ tsp. baking powder
- 1 tsp. vanilla extract
- 3 eggs

Directions:

1. Preheat the oven to 350°F. Prepare a muffin tray.
2. Meanwhile, mix flour, baking powder, cocoa powder, and Erythritol in a bowl. Add in heavy cream, vanilla, and eggs. Mix well.
3. Add in chocolate chips.
4. Scoop just the right amount of the batter into the muffin tray.
5. Place inside the oven and bake for 20 minutes.
6. Let cool before serving.

48. Fat Head Bagel

Ingredients:

- 1 ½ cup mozzarella cheese
- 1/8 cup cream cheese
- ¾ cup coconut or almond flour
- 1 teaspoon baking powder
- 1 egg
- Water

Directions:

1. Preheat the oven to 400F. Grease baking sheet with parchment paper. Set aside.
2. In a microwavable bowl, put mozzarella cheese and cream cheese. Mix well. Microwave for 30 seconds.
3. In a separate bowl, combine baking powder and flour.
4. Pour flour mixture into cheeses mixture. Place inside the microwave oven and bake for 30 seconds until elastic. Knead with the hand.
5. Divide into equal portions and roll into a ball. Layer on the baking sheet.
6. Brush balls with oil. Place inside the oven and bake for 15 minutes. Serve.

Spiced Dark Chocolate Bagel. Add ½ to 1 teaspoon of white pepper in Step 4. Bake.

In a saucepan, melt about 2 ounces of dark chocolate. Drizzle over or lightly dip the top of the bagel into the melted chocolate.

Note: Dark chocolate is allowed in Keto diet. However, check the nutritional facts of the brand you are using. Some chocolate compounds may use ingredients that are high in carbohydrates. Use dark chocolates that are about 70% cacao solid.

49. Cheesy Jalapeno Bagel

Ingredients:

- 1 ½ cup mozzarella cheese
- 1/8 cup cream cheese
- ¾ cup coconut or almond flour
- 1 teaspoon baking powder
- 1 cup cheddar cheese
- ½ cup jalapeno pepper
- 1 egg
- Water

Directions:

1. Preheat the oven to 400F. Grease baking sheet with parchment paper. Set aside.
2. In a microwavable bowl, put mozzarella cheese and cream cheese. Mix well. Microwave for 30 seconds.
3. In a separate bowl, combine baking powder and flour.
4. Pour flour mixture into cheeses mixture. Place inside the microwave oven and bake for 30 seconds until elastic. Knead with the hand.
5. Divide into equal portions and roll into a ball. Layer on the baking sheet.
6. Spread cheddar cheese and jalapeno pepper on top.
7. Brush balls with oil. Place inside the oven and bake for 15 minutes. Serve.

50. Cinnamon-Flavored Bagel

Ingredients:

- 1 ½ cup mozzarella cheese
- 1/8 cup cream cheese
- ¾ cup coconut flour
- 1 teaspoon cinnamon powder
- 1 teaspoon baking powder
- 1 egg
- water

Directions:

1. Preheat the oven to 400F. Grease baking sheet with parchment paper. Set aside.
2. In a microwavable bowl, put mozzarella cheese and cream cheese. Mix well. Microwave for 30 seconds.
3. In a separate bowl, combine baking powder, cinnamon powder, and flour.
4. Pour flour mixture into cheeses mixture. Place inside the microwave oven and bake for 30 seconds until elastic. Knead with the hand.
5. Divide into equal portions and roll into a ball. Layer on the baking sheet.
6. Brush balls with oil. Place inside the oven and bake for 15 minutes. Serve.

51. Dark Choco Bagel

Ingredients:

- 1 ½ cup mozzarella cheese
- 1/8 cup cream cheese
- ¾ cup coconut or almond flour
- 1 teaspoon baking powder
- ½ teaspoon of white pepper
- 1 egg
- Water
- ½ cup dark chocolate

Directions:

1. Preheat the oven to 400F. Grease baking sheet with parchment paper. Set aside.
2. In a microwavable bowl, put mozzarella cheese and cream cheese. Mix well. Microwave for 30 seconds.
3. In a separate bowl, combine baking powder, white pepper, and flour.
4. Pour flour mixture into cheeses mixture. Place inside the microwave oven and bake for 30 seconds until elastic. Knead with the hand.
5. Divide into equal portions and roll into a ball. Layer on the baking sheet.
6. Brush balls with oil. Place inside the oven and bake for 15 minutes. Serve.
7. In a saucepan, melt dark chocolate. Drizzle over bagel or dip.

Chapter 4 – Keto Cookies, Crackers, and Breadsticks

52. Sugar Lemon Cookies

Ingredients:

- ¼ cup almond flour
- 1 cup Erythritol sweetener
- ¼ cup flax meal
- 1 tsp. baking powder
- ¼ cup oat fiber
- 1-2 cups Erythitol sweetener
- ¼ cup coconut flour
- ¼ cup water
- 1 tbsp. vanilla extract
- ¾ tsp. cider vinegar
- 1/8 tsp. salt
- 2 large eggs
- 1 cup extra-virgin olive oil
- 6 lemons, zested and juiced

Directions:

1. Preheat the oven to 350°F. Line a baking sheet with parchment paper.
2. Combine the oat fiber, coconut and almond flours, and flax meal. Mix well. Add all other ingredients.
3. Knead until you get a dough that's slightly sticky.
4. Roll out the dough. Cut the dough with a cookie cutter and place on the baking sheet. Sprinkle Erythritol on top.
5. Bake for 12 minutes.

6. Meanwhile, mix lemon juice and sweetener in a bowl. A slightly thick consistency must be achieved.
7. Once cookies are cooled, spread icing over cookies. Refrigerate for a few minutes before serving.

53. Chocolate Cookies (Flourless)

Ingredients:

- 1 cup dark chocolate chips, sugar-free
- 1 cup coconut flakes
- ¾ cup walnuts, chopped
- ¼ cup coconut oil
- 4 tbsp. butter, softened
- 2 tbsp. Swerve sweetener
- 4 egg yolks

Directions:

1. Preheat the oven to 350°F (180°C). Line a baking sheet with parchment paper.
2. Add the oil, butter, egg yolks, and Swerve in a large bowl. Mix together well. Then, add the chocolate chips, walnuts, and coconut.
3. Put a spoonful of the batter on the baking sheet. Repeat until everything is in the sheet. You should get 18 pieces.
4. Bake for 15 minutes or until the cookies turn golden brown.

54. Cauliflower Bread Sticks

Serves: 12

Fat: about 5g Carbohydrates: about 74g

Protein: about 6g

Ingredients:

- 3 ½ cups dry cauliflower rice
- 1 ½ cup of mozzarella cheese or a combination of cheeses
- 1 egg
- Salt and pepper
- Two tablespoons Fresh parsley or basil, chopped finely
- Pinch of garlic powder

Direction:

1. Preheat oven to 225C (450F). Grease a baking sheet and line it with parchment paper.
2. Melt the cheese in the microwave.
3. Add the cauliflower rice and mix thoroughly. Add the egg and the rest of the ingredients.
4. Turn over the cauliflower-cheese mixture on the prepared baking sheet. Press it flat up to ¼" thick. Cut the sheet in slices using the pizza cutter or a sharp knife.
5. Bake in the oven for 15 to 20 minutes.

55. Raspberry Cookies

Ingredients:

- 4 oz. raspberries, chopped
- 1 ¼ cups almond flour
- ¼ cup coconut flour
- ½ cup Erythritol sweetener
- 1 tbsp. ghee, melted
- 1 tsp. vanilla extract
- 1 tsp. baking powder
- 1 medium egg

Directions:

1. Preheat the oven to 350°F (180°C).
2. Mix the flours, Erythritol, and baking powder until well-combined. Then, mix in the raspberries. Combine well.
3. Whip the vanilla and egg together. Slowly add the ghee while continuing to whisk.
4. Add the wet mixture to the bowl of the dry mixture and mix until you form a dough.
5. Divide into 10 and roll into balls. Place on a lined baking sheet and flatten with your palm.
6. Bake for 10-12 minutes. Rotate the tray halfway through baking. Let the cookies cool before serving

56. Basic Sugar Cookies

Ingredients:

- 1 cup extra-virgin olive oil
- 1 cup Erythritol sweetener
- ¼ cup oat fiber
- ¼ cup coconut flour
- ¼ cup almond flour
- ¼ cup flax meal
- ¼ cup water
- 1 tbsp. vanilla extract
- 1 tsp. baking powder
- ¾ tsp. cider vinegar
- 1/8 tsp. salt
- 2 large eggs

Directions:

1. Preheat the oven to 350°F (180°C). Line a baking sheet with parchment paper.
2. Combine the oat fiber, coconut and almond flours, and flax meal. Mix well, then add in all the other ingredients. Knead until you get a dough that's slightly sticky.
3. Roll out the dough until it's ¼-inch thick. Cut the dough with a cookie cutter and place the cookies on the baking sheet. Sprinkle extra Erythritol on top.
4. Bake for 8-12 minutes or until done.

57. Cheesy Garlic Breadsticks

Ingredients:

- 1 cup almond flour
- 3 tablespoons flaxseed meal
- 2 tablespoons coconut flour
- 2 teaspoons baking powder
- ½ teaspoon xanthan gum, optional but recommended
- 1/2 teaspoon garlic powder
- Salt and pepper
- 1/4 cup melted butter
- 2 eggs
- 1 cup mozzarella cheese
- 1 teaspoon minced garlic
- 2 tablespoons butter, softened
- 1/3 cup cheddar cheese

Directions:

1. Preheat the oven to 200C or 400F for at least 10 minutes.
2. Combine all the dry ingredients in a bowl.
3. Melt the mozzarella in the microwave for a minute. Stir in the dry ingredients. Heat for another minute.
4. Stir until the mixture cools down. Add the eggs and the melted butter. Mix by hand or by a spatula.
5. Place between two sheets of parchment paper and roll into ¼" thick. Remove the top parchment. Prick holes on the dough with a fork.
6. Transfer the flat dough to a greased baking sheet. Slice to desired size using a knife or a pizza cutter.
7. Bake in the oven for about 12 minutes. Meanwhile, mix the last three ingredients.

8. Remove the bread from the oven. Spread the garlic-butter mixture on top. Return to the oven and cook for another 5 to 7 minutes.

58. Walnut Cookies

Ingredients:

- 1 cup walnuts, ground
- ½ cup Erythritol sweetener
- ¼ cup coconut flour
- 8 tbsp. butter, softened
- 1 tsp. vanilla extract
- 1 tsp. nutmeg ground

Directions:

1. Preheat the oven to 325°F (165°C). Prepare two baking sheets and line with parchment paper.
2. Mix all the ingredients together except for the butter. Once combined, mix in the butter until your form a soft dough.
3. Divide the dough into 16 and form into balls.
4. Place the balls onto the baking sheet and flatten.
5. Bake for 13 minutes. Let the cookies cool to firm up.

Sandwiches

59. Anchovies and Tomatoes in Lettuce Wraps

Makes 2 servings, recommended serving size: 3 wraps

- 6 pieces, large butter lettuce leaves, rinsed, spun-dried, chilled well prior to use

For filling

- 1 tsp.capers in brine, lightly drained
- 1 tsp. fresh chives, minced
- 1 tsp. red wine vinegar
- 1 tsp. yellow mustard
- ⅛tsp. fish sauce
- 1 can, 2 oz. anchovy fillets in olive oil, low-sodium, drained well, roughly chopped
- ½ cup Asian or Mexican turnip, peeled, julienned
- ½ cup cashew nuts, freshly roasted on dry pan, unseasoned, roughly chopped, optional
- ¼ pound ripe cherry or grape tomatoes, quartered
- sea salt, only if needed
- white pepper, to taste

Directions:

1. <u>To prepare filling</u>: place ingredients into mixing bowl. Toss well to combine. Chill until ready to use. Divide into 6 equal portions.
2. <u>To prepare cucumber halves</u>: brush cut sides of avocado with equal amounts of lemon juice. Chill well prior to use.
3. <u>To assemble</u>: spoon equal portions of shrimp salad into prepared cucumber halves. Place on plates. Serve.

60. Cheese Steamed Pork Sliders

1 piece, large cucumber, sliced into 6 pieces ¼-inch thick medallions

For meatballs

- 1 piece, medium white/yellow onion, minced
- ½ pound lean ground pork
- Pinch red pepper flakes
- sea salt, only if needed
- white pepper, to taste
- ½ cup Colby Jack cheese, shredded, divided
- yellow mustard
- water, for steaming

Directions:

1. <u>To make meatballs</u>: half-fill steaming pot with water. Set over high heat. Secure lid. Boil water.
2. Place ground pork, onion, and red pepper flakes into mixing bowl. Season lightly with salt and pepper. Divide equally into 6 meatballs. Stuff each meatball into 3-ounce ramekins (or any similar sized steamer-safe cookware.)
3. Place ramekins on steam basket/tray. Steam burgers for 30 minutes.
4. Carefully remove steam basket from pot. Add equal portions of cheese on top of each burger. Return steam basket to pot. Secure lid. Steam for another 5 minutes. Turn off heat. Let burgers rest undisturbed for 10 minutes.

5. Carefully remove each burger from ramekins. Discard cooking juices.
6. <u>To assemble</u>: spread small amount of mustard on cucumber base. Place 1 cheeseburger on top. Top off with another cucumber medallion. Secure with toothpick if necessary. Repeat step until all burgers are stacked.
7. Place 3 sliders on plate. Serve.

62. Pepperoni on Tomato Bread

Ingredients:

- 2 pieces, large fresh, green tomatoes, sliced horizontally to make 4 ½-inch thick disks, mince remaining pieces

For sausages

- 4 slices, large classic or turkey pepperoni, rinds removed
- 4 slices, large classic or cracked black pepper salami, rinds removed
- 1 tsp. apple cider vinegar

For salsa

- 1 Tbsp. lemon juice, freshly squeezed
- 1 pinch, generous fresh cilantro, minced
- 2 pieces, large fresh ripe tomato, deseeded, minced
- 1 piece bird's eye chili, minced
- ½ piece, small shallot, minced
- 1 piece, small garlic clove, minced
- salt and black pepper, to taste

Directions:

1. <u>To make salsa</u>: combine ingredients in mixing bowl, including minced green tomatoes. Mix well. Taste. Adjust seasoning, if needed. Chill well prior to serving. Divide into equal portions.
2. <u>To cook sausages</u>: pour apple cider vinegar into skillet set over high heat . Cook salami and pepperoni slices until

only heated through, or fat in sausages turn transparent. Drain well.

3. <u>To assemble</u>: stack equal amounts of pepperoni and salami on 2 tomato slices. Top off with remaining tomatoes. Secure with toothpick, if needed. Serve with salsa on side.

63. Black Caraway Bread Sticks

Ingredients:

- 1 tablespoon black caraway seeds, add more if desired
- coconut oil for greasing

Bread

- 4 pieces large eggs, whisked
- 4 tablespoons ghee, add more for brushing
- 4 cups almond flour, add more for kneading if needed
- 1 teaspoon sea salt

Directions:

1. Preheat oven to 350°F/175°C. Line 2 baking sheets with aluminum foil; lightly grease with oil.
2. Combine bread ingredients in a bowl; mix until dough comes together. Turn out dough on lightly floured surface; knead until elastic and no longer sticks to your hands, adding more flour as needed. Rest dough for 5 minutes covered with saran wrap.
3. Turn out dough; roll into a log and divide into 18 balls. Roll each out into bread sticks about ½ inch thick and 6 inches long. Place sticks on baking sheets with spaces in between.
4. Brush *ghee* on top of each stick; sprinkle caraway seeds on top. Bake for 10 to 12 minutes. Remove baking sheets from oven; set on cake rack to cool. Serve.

64. Grain-Free Raisin Bread

Ingredients:

- 8 tablespoons coconut butter, add more for greasing
- 2 tablespoons lime juice, fresh squeezed
- 6 pieces large eggs, whisked
- 2 teaspoons cinnamon powder
- 2 teaspoons nutmeg powder
- 2 teaspoons baking soda
- 2 teaspoons vanilla extract
- 1 cup almond flour
- ½ cup raisins
- ½ cup sultanas
- Pinch, generous sea salt
- water for soaking

Directions:

1. Soak raisins and sultanas in water until double in size. Drain well.
2. Preheat oven to 350°F/175°C. Line an 11" x 7" x 2" loaf tin with parchment paper with long overhangs at the sides. Lightly grease with coconut butter.
3. Mix ingredients, including raisins and sultanas in bowl until just combined. Pour batter into loaf tin; bake for 45 to 50 minutes, or until bread crests over loaf tins.
4. Bake for another 20 minutes loosely tented with aluminum foil. Remove loaf tins from oven; set on cake racks. Cool completely before slicing. Serve.

65. Top Heavy Bread

Ingredients:

Toppings, optional

- 1 tablespoon heaping blanched almond slivers
- 1 tablespoon heaping pine nuts, chopped
- ½ teaspoon heaping sesame seeds
- ½ teaspoon heaping shelled roasted pumpkin seeds
- Pinch, generous garlic flakes
- Dash dried basil, shredded
- Dash dried thyme, shredded

Bread loaf

- 5 pieces large eggs, whisked
- 4 tablespoons coconut oil, reserve some for greasing
- 1 tablespoon coconut vinegar
- 1 cup almond flour
- 1 cup coconut flour
- ¼ cup tapioca flour
- 1 teaspoon baking soda
- ¼ teaspoon sea salt

Directions:

1. Preheat oven to 350°F/175°C. Line 8½" x 4½" x 2½" loaf tin with aluminum foil; lightly grease with coconut oil.
2. Mix bread loaf ingredients in a bowl until just combined; pour batter into loaf tin. Sprinkle in desired toppings.
3. Bake for 30 to 40 minutes, or until toothpick inserted in center comes out clean. Remove from heat; cool bread in

tin for 2 hours. Remove from tins; set bread on cake rack to completely. Slice. Serve.

66. Almond Bread Twists

Ingredients:

- 2 drops almond extract
- 2 cups almond flour, finely-milled
- ½ cup chilled coconut butte
- ½ cup honey-roasted almond
- 1 tablespoon all-purpose flour
- 1 egg, whisked lightly
- oil for frying
- cold water only if needed
- powdered sugar for dusting

Directions:

1. Process butter into finely milled flour until latter resembles breadcrumbs. Stir in all-purpose flour, almond extract, egg, and honey-roasted almonds until dough comes together.
2. If dough doesn't form, add a teaspoon of water at a time. Mix well after each addition. Turn out dough on lightly floured surface; knead until elastic. Equally divide dough into 8 balls; roll each one out into 10-inch long ribbons
3. Fold lengthwise once and roll out again to flatten; repeat step 5 times to make bread flaky. Roll out bread into a ribbon one final time; twist twice. Place on baking sheet lined with parchment paper. Repeat steps until all breadsticks are rolled and twisted; chill well before cooking.
4. Half fill deep fryer with oil; set over medium heat. When oil becomes slightly smoky, slide in a few breadsticks at a

time; cook until golden brown. Place cooked bread on platter lined with paper towels.

5. Place 2 pieces of breadsticks on plate; dust with small amount of powdered sugar. Cool slightly before serving.

67. Chia Seed Bread

Ingredients:

- coconut oil for greasing
- 1 teaspoon chia seeds, whole

Dry ingredients

- 3 cups almond flour
- $^1/_3$ cup arrowroot powder
- ½ tablespoon chia seed, coarsely ground
- 1½ teaspoons baking soda
- ½ teaspoon sea salt

Wet ingredients

- 6 pieces medium eggs, whisked
- ¾ cup coconut cream
- ½ cup butter, melted
- 1½ teaspoons coconut vinegar

Directions:

1. Preheat oven to 350°F/175°C. Lightly grease an 8½" x 4½" x 2½" loaf tin.
2. Combine dry ingredients in a bowl; make well in center. Pour in wet ingredients; stir until just combined. Pour into prepared loaf tin. Sprinkle whole chia seeds on top.
3. Bake for 30 to 35 minutes, or until toothpick inserted in center comes out clean. Remove pan from oven; set on cake rack to cool slightly. Remove bread from tin. Cool completely before slicing. Serve.

68. Coconut with Chestnut Bread

Ingredients:

- 2 tablespoons coconut flakes, divided
- coconut oil for greasing

Dry ingredients

- 3 cups almond meal
- 2 cups chestnut flour
- ½ cup, packed roasted chestnuts, diced
- $^2/_3$ cup arrowroot flour
- 1½ teaspoons sea salt

Wet ingredients

- 14 pieces large eggs, yolks and whites separated
- 2 tablespoons stevia
- $^2/_3$ cup coconut cream
- $^2/_3$ cup coconut oil

Directions:

1. Preheat oven to 325°F/160°C. Line 2 7½" x 3½" x 2" loaf tins with parchment paper; lightly grease with coconut oil.
2. Combine dry ingredients in a bowl; make well in center. Except for the egg whites, pour in all the wet ingredients. Mix batter until just combined.
3. Whisk egg whites in another bowl until stiff peaks form; gently fold in into bread batter. Pour equal portions of batter into loaf tins; top off with coconut flakes.

4. Bake for 40 to 45 minutes, or until toothpick inserted in center comes out clean. Cover tins with aluminum foil if bread tops are browning too fast.
5. Cool in tins for 2 hours; set on cake rack to cool completely before slicing. Serve plain or toasted with spread of choice.

69. Totally Vegan Pizza

Ingredients:

- 1 slice pizza loaf, lightly toasted
- 1 tablespoon tomato sauce
- 1 tablespoon cashew cheese
- ½ tablespoon shallot, julienned
- ½ tablespoon red bell pepper, julienned
- Dash of red pepper flakes
- Pinch of black pepper
- extra virgin oil, for drizzling

Directions:

1. Spread tomato sauce on one side of bread. Layer shallot and bell pepper slices on top. Drizzle in cashew cheese and olive oil; season lightly with black pepper.
2. Heat pizza slice in toaster oven until warmed through. Serve.

70. Chestnut and Coconut Bread

Ingredients:

- 1 tablespoon coconut flakes, sweetened, divided
- coconut oil for greasing
- butter for spreading, optional

Dry ingredients

- 4 cups almond meal, finely milled
- $2/3$ cup tapioca flour
- 1 cup chestnut flour
- 1½ tsp. sea salt
- 1 cup roasted shelled chestnuts, minced

Wet ingredients

- $2/3$ cup coconut milk
- 2 drops stevia
- $2/3$ cup coconut oil
- 14 large eggs, yolks and whites separated

Coconut butter

- 6 cups coconut flakes, unsweetened

Directions:

1. Preheat the oven to 325 degrees °F. Lightly grease loaf tins with coconut oil.

2. Process coconut flakes in a blender. Process for 5 minutes with 30 second intervals or until you achieve a buttery consistency. Store coconut butter in an airtight container.
3. Meanwhile, beat egg whites. Set aside.
4. Put almond meal, tapioca flour, chestnut flour, and salt in a food processor. Process until powdery. Pour in a mixing bowl. Make a well in the center.
5. In a separate bowl, combine coconut milk, stevia, coconut oil, and roasted chestnuts. Mix well. Fold in egg whites.
6. Divide batter into loaf tins. Dust coconut flakes on top of each loaf tin. Bake for 40 minutes. Remove from heat.
7. Cool bread loaves for 2 hours. At room temperature, cool completely before slicing into thick pieces. Serve

71. Keto-Friendly Bread with Olives and Onions

Ingredients:

- 2 slices Ketogenic-friendly read such as **Error! eference source not found.**, toasted
- 2 large garlic cloves, peeled
- ⅛ teaspoon extra virgin olive oil

Vegetable spread

- 1 large black olive in oil, pitted, thinly sliced
- 1 large green olive in brine, pitted, thinly sliced
- 1 large roasted red pepper in oil, julienned
- 1 teaspoon apple cider vinegar
- ¼ cup cucumber, deseeded, julienned
- ⅛ cup shallot, minced
- Pinch of sea salt
- Pinch of black pepper to taste

Directions:

1. Preheat oven toaster.
2. Rub garlic cloves on both sides of toasted bread. Mix vegetable spread ingredients in a small bowl. Taste; adjust seasoning if needed.
3. Spread on bread slices. Place bread into oven toaster to warm through. Remove from heat. Drizzle in olive oil just before serving.

72. Asparagus and Squash Flowers Pizza

Ingredients:

- ½ any plant-based-approved dough such as sourdough dough

For the topping

- 6 asparagus spears, sliced into 1-inch long slivers
- 12 squash flowers, petals only, torn
- 1 tsp. capers in brine
- 1 can button mushrooms
- ¼ tsp. garlic salt, vegan-safe
- extra virgin oil
- black pepper, to taste

Directions:

1. Preheat oven to 430°F or 220°C. Lightly grease a 10-inch pizza tray with olive oil.
2. Place dough on pizza tray. Using your fingers and knuckles, stretch dough out so it covers entire surface of pizza tray. Season dough with garlic salt.
3. Layer on the asparagus slivers, button mushrooms and capers.
4. Spread squash flowers on top and season well with olive oil and black pepper.
5. Bake pizza for 8 to 10 minutes, or until flowers brown a little and crust crisps up.
6. Remove pizza tray from oven and place on cooling rack for at least 3 minutes prior to slicing.
7. Slice pizza into 6 generous portions or 8 smaller slices. Serve.

73. Chia Seed Bread

Ingredients:

- 2 slices Chia Seed Bread, toasted
- 2 large garlic cloves, peeled
- ⅛ teaspoon extra virgin olive oil

Tapenade

- 6 large black olives in oil, pitted, minced
- 2 tablespoons golden raisins, soaked in water, minced
- 1 tablespoon capers in brine, drained, minced
- 1 tablespoon fresh parsley, minced
- 1 tablespoon lime juice, freshly squeezed
- ¼ tablespoon fresh thyme, minced
- Pinch of sea salt
- Pinch of white pepper

Directions:

1. Preheat oven toaster.
2. Rub garlic cloves on both sides of toasted bread. Mix tapenade ingredients in a small bowl. Taste; adjust seasoning if needed.
3. Spread on bread slices. Place bread into the oven toaster to warm through. Remove from heat. Drizzle in olive oil just before serving.

74. Psyllium Husk & Coconut Flour Loaf

Ingredients:

- 1 cup coconut flour
- ¾ cup warm water
- ½ cup olive oil
- ¼ cup coconut oil, melted
- 6 tbsp. psyllium husks, ground finely
- 1 ½ tsp. baking soda
- ¾ tsp. sea salt
- 2 large eggs + 2 cups egg whites

Directions:

1. Preheat the oven to 350°F (180°C). Prepare an 8x4-inch loaf tin lined with parchment paper.
2. Mix all the ingredients together until well-combined.
3. Bake the bread for 45-55 minutes until edges turn brown or until it passes the toothpick test.
4. Let the bread cool for 15 minutes before removing from the loaf tin and slicing.

75. Flatbread

Ingredients:

- ¾ cup mozzarella, melted
- 2 tbsp. almond flour
- 1 tbsp. cream cheese, melted
- 1 tbsp. basil
- 1 tbsp. garlic powder
- 1 egg

Directions:

1. Preheat your oven to 350°F (180°C) and prepare a greased ramekin.
2. Mix all the ingredients together except for the garlic powder.
3. Divide the mixture into 8 and flatten each portion on a baking sheet. Sprinkle the garlic on top of the bread.
4. Bake for 20 minutes or until edges start to brown.

76. Buttery Garlic Bread

Ingredients:

- 7 oz. full-fat cream cheese, softened
- 2 garlic cloves, crushed + 1 clove, crushed for the glaze
- ¼ cup butter, melted for the glaze
- 1 cup almond flour
- 3 tbsp. psyllium husks
- 3 tbsp. coconut flour
- 1 tsp. salt
- 6 eggs

Directions:

1. Preheat your oven to 350°F (180°C). Line a baking sheet with parchment paper.
2. Beat the cream cheese and 2 crushed garlic cloves together. Then, add the eggs one at a time while continuing to whisk.
3. Add in the rest of the ingredients and fold gently until you form a dough.
4. Shape the dough into a loaf on the baking sheet. Set aside.
5. Mix the butter and garlic to make the glaze. Brush ¼ of the garlic butter on the dough. Save the rest for later.
6. Bake for 20 minutes. Halfway through baking, score the top of the bread to cook evenly. The bread should turn golden brown once done.
7. Cut the bread into 14 slices and drizzle the rest of the glaze on top before serving.

77. Cheese & Bacon Bread

Ingredients:

- 7 oz. bacon, driced
- 1 ½ cups almond flour
- 1 cup cheddar, grated
- 1/3 cup sour cream
- 4 tbsp. butter, melted
- 1 tbsp. baking powder
- 2 eggs

Directions:

1. Preheat your oven to 300°F (150°C). Grease and line a loaf tin with parchment paper.
2. Cook the bacon in a pan until crispy. Set aside.
3. Mix the baking powder and flour in a bowl. In a separate bowl, whisk the eggs and sour cream until smooth.
4. Add the egg mixture to the flour mixture. Mix until well-combined.
5. Then, mix in the melted butter. Finally, fold the cheese and bacon into the batter.
6. Transfer the batter to the loaf tin. Bake for 45-50 minutes or until the bread passes the toothpick test.
7. Let the bread cool to firm up before slicing.

78. Dinner Rolls

Ingredients:

- 1/3 cup coconut flour
- ¼ cup almond flour
- ¼ cup ghee, melted
- ¼ cup water
- ¼ cup psyllium husk powder
- 2 tsp. olive oil
- 1 tsp. baking soda
- 1 tsp. baking powder
- 4 eggs

Directions:

1. Preheat your oven to 350°F (180°C) and prepare a lined baking sheet.
2. Mix all the dry ingredients together until well-combined.
3. In a separate bowl, combine the wet ingredients and mix well.
4. Combine the wet and dry ingredients. Mix well to form a soft dough. Let it rest for about 5 minutes to firm up.
5. Divide the dough into 9 equal portions and form into balls.
6. Place them on the baking sheet and bake for about 25-30 minutes. Reduce the temperature to 300°F (150°C) for the last 10 minutes of baking.

79. Irish Soda Bread

Ingredients:

- 1 oz. raisins
- 1 ¼ cups almond flour
- 2 tbsp. coconut flour
- 2 tbsp. sour cream
- ½ tbsp. Swerve sweetener
- ½ tbsp. apple cider vinegar
- 1 tsp. baking powder
- 1 tsp. baking soda
- 1/8 tsp. kosher salt
- 2 large eggs, whisked

Directions:

1. Preheat your oven to 350°F (180°C). Grease an 8-inch cast iron pan.
2. Add all the dry ingredients and the raisins in a bowl. Mix well to remove any clumps.
3. Then, add the remaining ingredients and mix until well-combined.
4. Place the dough in the greased pan and shape into an oval loaf. Score the top of the bread with an X. Sprinkle with extra Swerve.
5. Bake for about 25-28 minutes or until it becomes golden brown and passes the toothpick test.
6. Completely cool the bread before removing from the pan and slicing.

80. Microwaveable Hamburger Bun

Ingredients:

- 3 tbsp. almond flour
- 1 ½ tbsp. olive oil
- ½ tsp. baking powder
- 1 egg

Directions:

1. Mix the flour and baking powder well to remove clumps. Then, mix in the egg and oil.
2. Beat the mixture well until well-blended. You can use any small microwaveable bowl to cook the bread.
3. Microwave the bread for 90 seconds on high.
4. Cut the hamburger bun and use as you wish.

81. Naan Bread

Ingredients:

- 1 cup water, boiling
- ½ cup coconut flour
- 2 tbsp. ghee, melted
- 2 tbsp. whole psyllium husks
- ¼ tsp. salt
- ¼ tsp. baking powder
- 1 egg

Directions:

1. Mix all the ingredients together until you form a dough. Knead, then refrigerate for an hour.
2. Divide the dough into 8 portions. Roll each portion into balls and flatten into desired shape.
3. Cook the bread over medium heat in a cast iron skillet. Cook each side for about 2 minutes or until it starts to become golden brown and puffy.

82. Pumpkin Bread Loaf

Ingredients:

- 2 cups blanched almond flour
- ¾ cup Erythritol sweetener
- ¼ cup pumpkin puree
- ½ cup coconut flour
- 1/3 cup butter, melted
- ¼ cup pumpkin seeds
- 2 tsp. pumpkin spice
- 2 tsp. baking powder, gluten-free
- ¼ tsp. sea salt
- 4 large eggs, beaten

Directions:

1. Preheat your oven to 350°F (180°C). Prepare a 9x5-inch loaf tin lined with parchment paper.
2. Combine the flours, sweetener, pumpkin spice, salt, and baking powder in a bowl. Mix until well-combined.
3. Then, add in the puree, eggs, and butter. Mix everything well.
4. Pour the batter into the loaf tin and smoothen the top. Sprinkle with the seeds and press lightly.
5. Bake for 50 minutes up to an hour or until it passes the toothpick test.
6. Cool it completely before taking out of the pan. Slice into 12 pieces.

83. Pork Rind Bread

Ingredients:

- 8 oz. cream cheese
- 2 cups mozzarella, grated
- ¼ cup parmesan, grated
- 1 cup pork rinds, crushed
- 1 tbsp. baking powder
- 3 large eggs

Directions:

1. Preheat your oven to 375°F (190°C). Prepare a 12x17-inch baking sheet lined with parchment paper.
2. Melt the mozzarella and cream cheese together and mix well.
3. Add the pork rinds, parmesan, baking powder, and egg. Mix until well-combined.
4. Spread the batter onto the baking sheet.
5. Bake for 15-20 minutes until the top browns lightly.
6. Let it cool for a few minutes before removing from the pan. Slice into 12 pieces equally.

84. Flaxseed Tortilla Wraps

Yields: 6 tortillas

Ingredients:

- ¼ cup mozzarella, grated
- 6 tbsp. milled flax seeds
- 6 tbsp. water
- ¼ tsp. xanthan gum
- 3 large eggs

Directions:

1. Mix all the ingredients together using a food processor until well-combined
2. Heat some oil or butter in a pan over medium heat. It's best to use an 8-inch pan.
3. Spoon 2 tbsp. of the batter into the pan. Swirl around to fill the pan. Let the top bubble, then flip the wrap over. Continue to cook until the other side turns brown.

85. Basic Biscuits

Ingredients:

- 1 ¼ cups almond flour
- 1/3 cup mozzarella, grated
- 1/3 cup sour cream
- 5 tbsp. butter, melted
- ½ tsp. sea salt
- ½ tsp. baking powder
- 2 large eggs

Directions:

1. Preheat your oven to 400°F (200°C). Grease an 8-piece muffin tin with some cooking spray.
2. Mix all the ingredients together until well-combined.
3. Equally distribute the batter into 8 cups of the muffin tin. They should only be 2/3 full.
4. Bake for 10-15 minutes until the tops turn light golden. Let them cool for 3 minutes.

86. Cheesy Garlic Biscuits

Ingredients:

- 1 cup blanched almond flour
- ¾ cup parmesan, grated
- ½ cup coconut oil, melted
- 1/3 cup coconut flour
- 1 tbsp. dried parsley
- 2 tsp. baking powder, gluten-free
- 6 garlic cloves, minced
- 5 large eggs

Directions:

1. Preheat your oven to 350°F (180°C) and prepare a lined baking sheet.
2. Mix all the dry ingredients in a mixing bowl. Then, stir in the wet ingredients. Mix well and let it sit for a few minutes and let it thicken.
3. Place a tablespoonful of the batter onto your baking sheet. Shape it into a biscuit and flatten it lightly. Repeat until you use up all the batter. You should get 14 pieces.
4. Sprinkle extra parmesan on top if you prefer. Then, bake for 15-20 minutes or until the biscuits are golden brown and firm.

87. Yogurt Herbed Biscuits

Ingredients:

- 1 cup coconut flour
- ¼ cup plain yogurt
- 2 tsp. baking powder
- 2 tsp. fresh dill
- 1 tsp. onion powder
- A pinch of sea salt
- 1 egg, beaten

Directions:

1. Preheat your oven to 350°F (180°C). Line a baking sheet with parchment paper.
2. Mix all the dry ingredients until well-combined. Then, fold in the egg and yogurt. Mix until you get a frothy and thick batter.
3. Scoop the batter onto the parchment paper dividing it into 6 portions equally.
4. Bake for 15 minutes until it turns golden brown. Let it cool for a bit to firm up.

88. Basic Almond Biscotti

Ingredients:

- ¼ cup + 2 tbsp. almond flour
- ¼ cup almonds, chopped
- 3 tbsp. butter, melted
- 2 tsp. Stevia sweetener
- ½ tsp. baking powder
- ½ tsp. vanilla extract
- 1 egg, beaten

Directions:

1. Preheat your oven to 350°F (180°C) and prepare a greased baking sheet.
2. Combine the flour, almonds, and baking powder together.
3. Mix in the butter, vanilla, Stevia, and egg. Continue to stir until you form a firm dough.
4. Create a 1-cm thick log with the dough. Slice the bread into 10 equal sizes.
5. Place the biscotti on the baking sheet and bake for 10 minutes.
6. Then, take the biscuits out of the oven and reduce the oven temperature to 325°F (170°C).
7. Turn the biscotti and bake for an additional 10-15 minutes or until they turn golden brown.

89. Caramel & Chocolate Biscotti

Ingredients:

- 2 ¼ cups almond flour
- ¼ cup pecans, toasted and chopped
- ¼ cup Stevia sweetener
- ¼ cup cold butter, cubed
- 2 tbsp. chocolate chips, sugar-free
- 2 tbsp. Erythritol sweetener
- 2 tbsp. coconut flour
- 1 tbsp. caramel coffee syrup, sugar-free
- ¾ tsp. baking powder
- ½ tsp. xanthan gum
- 1 egg

Directions:

1. Preheat your oven to 325°F (170°C) and prepare a greased baking sheet.
2. Mix all the ingredients together except for the butter, egg, and syrup. Continue mixing until well-combined.
3. Then, add a few cubes of the butter at a time while mixing. Make sure everything's well-blended before adding the syrup and egg. Mix until you form a dough.
4. Place the dough on a sheet of parchment paper. Then, form it into a loaf that's 2-inch thick and 10-inch long.
5. Transfer to the baking sheet and bake for 20 minutes.
6. Take out from the oven and reduce the oven temperature to 300°F (150°C).
7. Let the loaf cool for 30 minutes before slicing into 16 pieces. Then, place the slices back on the baking sheet with the cut-size down.
8. Bake for an additional 10 minutes. Cool completely before serving.

90. Pecan Bread Short Sticks/Crackers

Ingredients:

- 2 ¼ almond or coconut flour
- 1 cup butter, softened
- 1 cup cheddar cheese, grated
- ½ cup chopped toasted pecans
- ½ teaspoon each of salt and cayenne pepper

Directions:

1. Mix the butter and the cheese until well incorporated.
2. Fold in the toasted pecan.
3. In a separate bowl, mix the rest of the ingredients. Add half to the butter mixture. Mix by hand. Gradually add the remaining flour mixture to the butter. Knead until the dough achieves a texture of a shortbread.
4. Roll the dough into a log with a diameter of two inches. Wrap the logs with cling wrap and chill for 4 hours or overnight.
5. Grease a baking sheet and line with parchment paper. Preheat the oven to 350F (175C) for at least 10 minutes.
   If you want soft breadsticks, but hard on the outside, skip the preheating. Note: this applies only to breadsticks.
6. Slice the dough into ¼" rounds. Arrange on the baking sheet. For the breadsticks, roll the rounds into 1½-inch logs. Make sure that the diameter is at least ¼" thick.
7. Bake in the oven for 12 to 15 minutes. Cool in the pan for 1 minute before turning it over to a plate or cooling rack.
8. Sprinkle with some grated cheese before serving

Variations:

- ***Almond Breadsticks/Crackers****. Substitute the pecan with toasted almond. You may also use macadamia nuts or a combination of three.
- ***Herbed Sesame Breadsticks/Crackers.*** Substitute all or half of the pecana with toasted sesame seeds. Use rosemary, basil, oregano, parsley, or Italian seasoning instead of cayenne pepper.
- ***Seedy Breadsticks/Crackers.*** Substitute the pecan with sunflower seeds and sesame seeds.

91. Delicious Gluten-Free Breadsticks

Serves: 8

Fat: about 7g Carbohydrates: about 2g

Protein: about 4g

Ingredients:

- 3 tablespoons coconut oil or softened butter
- 3 tablespoons water
- 1/3 cup coconut or almond flour
- 1/3 cup arrowroot flour or flaxseed meal
- ½ teaspoon baking soda
- 1 ½ tablespoons of lime juice
- Pinch of salt
- 1 egg
- 1 tablespoon olive oil
- Finely Chopped herbs (optional)
- Sesame seeds (optional)
- Minced garlic (optional)

Directions:

1. Preheat the oven to 175C (350F) for at least 10 minutes.
2. Combine all ingredients in a bowl. Mix by hand or with an electric mixer until all ingredients are incorporated well.
3. Form into a bowl. Flatten the top and divide into 8 portions.
4. Roll each portion into logs with at least ½" diameter. Arrange on a greased baking sheet lined with parchment paper.

5. Brush the top with olive oil. Sprinkle top with herbs, garlic, and sesame seeds. Press the herbs to the dough.
6. Bake in the oven for 12 to 15 minutes or until golden brown.

92. Garlic Breadsticks

Ingredients:

- 4 cups almond flour
- 6 cup butter
- 1 teaspoon xanthan gum
- 2 eggs
- 1 teaspoon baking powder
- ½ teaspoon salt
- ½ cup boiling water
- 1 teaspoon garlic powder
- ¼ cup softened butter
- ½ tablespoon of toasted garlic bits, minced finely (optional)

Directions:

1. Preheat the oven to 200C or 400F for 10 minutes. Grease a baking sheet and line with parchment paper.
2. Mix all the dry ingredients except the garlic powder.
3. Melt the 6 tablespoons of butter and pour into the dry ingredients. Add the eggs. Mix using a spatula.
4. Pour the boiling water in the mixture. Mix with a spatula or by hand.
5. Form into a bowl and divide into 12 to 16 portions. Roll each portion into logs with at least ½" diameter. TIP: The dough is easier to roll with wet hands.
6. Arrange the sticks in the baking sheets. Bake for 15 minutes.
7. Meanwhile, mix the softened butter and garlic powder. Set aside.
8. Remove the breadsticks from the oven. Flip the sticks. Brush the new top with the garlic-butter mixture. Sprinkle with garlic bits. Press the bits on the dough.

9. Bake for another 5 minutes. Cool in the pan for a minute before transferring it to a jar or a serving platter.

93. Italian Breadsticks

Ingredients:

- 1 1/2 cups coconut or almond flour
- 2 1/2 cups mozzarella cheese, shredded
- ¾ cup cream cheese
- 2 large eggs
- 2 tablespoons Parmesan cheese, grated
- ½ teaspoon grated garlic or a pinch of garlic powder
- ½ teaspoon xanthan gum or 1 tablespoon of arrowroot or flaxseed flour
- 1 teaspoon deactivated yeast or nutritional yeast
- 2 teaspoons baking powder
- 1 teaspoon dried basil
- ¼ teaspoon parsley
- ¼ teaspoon rosemary
- Olive oil

Direction:

1. Preheat the oven to 400F (200C). Grease a baking sheet and line with parchment paper. Set aside.
2. Mix all the dry ingredients in a bowl.
3. Melt the mozzarella cheese and cream cheese in the microwave for 1 minute. Stir. Place back in the microwave and reheat for another minute. Stir to cool.
4. Stir in the fresh garlic and the eggs until the egg is incorporated. Sprinkle with Parmesan cheese.
5. Give a quick mix and add the dry ingredients. Mix to form a soft dough.
6. Turn over the dough to a kneading board. With wet or greased hands, knead the dough gently.

7. Form into a ball. Flatten it a little and divide into 12 or 16 portions. Roll each portion into sticks with at least ½" diameter. Arrange on the prepared baking sheet.
8. Bake for 12 minutes. Turn the sticks over and brush the top with olive oil. Bake for another 5 minutes.
9. Cool for a minute and transfer to a serving dish. Sprinkle with finely grated Parmesan or cheddar cheese. Serve with keto marinara sauce or garlic-butter.

TIP: This recipe can also be a good pizza crust. After flipping the crust, brush it with olive oil and top with choice of topping. Bake for 5 to 10 minutes. The temperature may be lowered depending on the toppings.

Tip for Crackers and Breadsticks

- All the dough recipes for the crackers and breadsticks, except those with fresh vegetables, can be frozen for two weeks. It would be good to double the dough and store the other portion for the next few days.
- All the rolled breadsticks and crackers can stay hard or crispy for three days to a week when kept in a tightly-sealed container.

Conclusion

Thank you again for purchasing this book.

This book has shared with you ketogenic recipes that can last you for more than 30 days. all are easy-to-prepare, delicious, and nutritious. You can just repeat some of the recipes for breakfast, lunch, dinner, and desserts and snacks since you have a wide selection to choose from.

May this cookbook serve as your guide to living the ketogenic lifestyle for the next 30 days and the rest of the days and months to come.

Invest more time in the kitchen to make your own meals, so that you will be able to save not just money but also your health.

Take pleasure in creating meal plans and collecting more ketogenic vegetarian recipes so that you can continue to enjoy the benefits of following this diet.

The next step is to try making your own recipes using ketogenic-safe ingredients.

Finally, if you enjoyed this book, then I'd like to ask you for a favor, would you be kind enough to leave a review for this book on Amazon? It'd be greatly appreciated!

Please leave a review for this book on Amazon!

Thank you and good luck!

49081555R00078

Made in the USA
Lexington, KY
20 August 2019